Target Fitness: How to stop unhealthy eating and overcome your addiction for food.

Casey.L.Clark

.

Table of content

Chapter1

What is unhealthy eating and why it is so Addictive

Unhealthy eating involves consuming food which are high in sugars, saturated and trans-fats, low fiber foods and high-sugar drinks,which most people feel they cannot do without,forgetting that such a poor diet can contribute to non-communicable diseases (NCDs) and other health problems. High intake of fast food and processed foods increases these health risks.

Food addiction can be defined as a constant obsession with what to eat, when to eat, and how to obtain more food; overeating behaviors; hiding or hoarding foods, secretive behaviors, and inability to stop overeating or continued eating. Food addiction is a psychological and emotional addiction to specific foods and substances. Even though it is not directly the same as a substance addiction, food activates the taste-reward and pleasurable regions of the brain are somewhat the same.

It's Addiction

If the brain notices that the amount of dopamine is too high, it begins removing dopamine receptors to make things balanced. When there are little receptors, more dopamine is required to reach the same effect, which causes people to start eating more junk food to reach the same level of reward as before.

“I consider junk food to be anything that doesn’t have any nutritional value,” says Komar. “They are your treat-type foods to have occasionally, but not all the time.”

What makes junk food taste so good?
You know junk food doesn’t make you feel your best, but why is it so hard to quit?

“This gets into the wonderful world of the science of food,” she explains. “Processed foods are mainly salt, sugar, fat and preservatives — all of which create a combination of different sensations in your mouth. Your brain is involved as well. Foods that rapidly vanish or ‘melt in your mouth’ signal to your brain that you’re not eating as much as you actually are. In other words, these foods literally tell your brain that you’re not full and you need more of the food. It sounds so good, but actually, you are not fueling your body, but burdening it to work very hard to metabolize junk food.”

It is also important to know that food companies invest a lot of time, money and resources into creating products that keep you coming back for more.

“Food companies will spend millions of money to discover the most satisfying level of junk food there is “Don't get caught in their traps.eating too much of an unhealthy thing, does not mean you lack self-control or will power; there is a highly competitive, secretive and successful food industry that exists only for one reason: to make junk food as addictive as possible so that we keep on eating.

It's not a surprise, of course, that food companies aim to give consumers what they want to optimize their profits, but the process of product development is actually quite sophisticated, relies on psychology and neuroscience, and is tested rigorously before it's aggressively and expertly marketed to us. For companies, the entire process is geared towards finding a particular food's "bliss point", which is the ratio of three nutrients: salt, sugar, and fat. These compounds trigger all our taste buds together, which further activate pleasure receptors in the brain.

The term "bliss point" was coined in the late 1990s by American market researcher and psychophysicist Howard Moskowitz. He defined it as "that sensory profile where you like food the most"; think Goldilocks quest for the perfect porridge — a food at its bliss point will make the eater feel that there is not too little or too much, but the "just right" amount of saltiness, sweetness, or richness (from the fat). This perfect point of snackability is what makes the eater reach out for more, more and more. Natural foods also have these three products, but not in the perfect "bliss point" ratio that will make our brains keep eating, independent of our hunger level.

"Junk foods specifically trigger our brain's "reward zone," the same area where drugs and alcohol act. Each time you eat sugar, your brain releases dopamine which is the happy hormone, and you feel good. In fact, food manufacturers spend millions to find the "bliss point"i.e the satisfactory point for each food,"These foods bypass our normal fullness mechanisms, which is why you could eat them all day and not feel full. Over time, your body becomes less sensitive to these foods, so you have to eat more just to get the same dopamine rush and satisfaction which makes you feel withdrawn if

.

you don't get it. It's like a designer drug in an easy-to-open package."

It's a very precise and well thought process, established to exploit our evolutionary systems' vulnerability to sugar, fat, and salt,
Technology has clearly outpaced biology now; even though we consume an unhealthy amount of salt, sugar and fat today, our brains remain evolutionarily designed to reward behaviors that procure these nutrients. "Simply put, our bodies are biologically wired to seek out high fat, high salt, high sugar foods – so-called hyper-palatable foods – and the corporations that feed us are profiting from those instincts, all the while putting our health at serious risk,"
Additionally..Food addicts become dependent upon the "good" feelings that are obtained from consuming certain foods, which often perpetuates a continued need to eat, even when not hungry. These behaviors generate a vicious cycle. As the food addict continues to pound upon foods that induce pleasurable feelings, they

often overindulge and eat beyond what is required for satiety.

Because of the ferocious cycle of food addiction and the detrimental consequences associated with this behavior, it is crucial that professional help is sought. If you or a loved one has been struggling with an addiction to food, consider the possibilities of a life free of this burden. You can find peace from an addiction to food by seeking the appropriate care and help you need.

Food addiction is likely the culmination of several factors that interplay in the overall cause of this disorder. A man or woman may develop an addiction as a result of biological, psychological, or social reasons. Biological causes that may influence the progression of this eating disorder might include hormonal imbalances, abnormalities in various brain structures, side effects from the use of certain medications, or having family members with this type of addiction issues.

It also might also be the result of psychological factors. Factors included in this category might include emotional or sexual abuse, being a victim or survivor of a traumatic event, having an inability to cope with negative situations, serious low-self esteem, or experiencing grief or loss.

Psychological factors such as these can influence an individual to use food as a coping mechanism to relieve the painful emotions that may have resulted. Lastly, there are social implications that may be involved with food addiction, including factors such as disturbances in family function, pressure from peers or society, social isolation, child abuse, lack of social support, and stressful life events.

Stress can also be a very important factor which causes the urge to eat lots of junk because when you are stressed out your whole body actually goes into a state of confusion.

An addiction to food can also be associated with other co-occurring disorders, such as eating disorders or substance abuse. Because food addiction is a complex mental health issue that can have serious complications if left untreated, it is highly recommended that professional help be sought to effectively heal from this disorder.

.

Chapter 2

Signs and symptoms of food addiction

This Eating Disorder can be noticed by numerous signs and symptoms. The following are possible symptoms of an addiction to food:

1.Taking in more food than one can physically tolerate
2.Eating to the point of feeling ill
3.Going out of your way to obtain certain foods
5.persistence to eat certain foods even if you are no longer hungry
6.Eating in secret, isolation totally away from people
7.Avoiding social interactions, relationships, or functions to spend time eating certain foods.
8.Finding it hard to function in a carccr or job due to decreased efficiency
9.Spending a significant amount of money on buying certain foods for binging purposes
10.Decreased energy, chronic fatigue
Difficulty concentrating

.

11.Sleep disorders, such as insomnia or oversleeping
12.Restlessness
13.Irritability
14.Headaches
15.Digestive disorders
16.Suicidal ideations because when you are isolated numerous sucidal thoughts tends to occur

*If you or your loved one has been experiencing any of these above symptoms as a result of food addiction, seek out professional help immediately to work through these pertinent issues.

Effects of Being a Food Addict

If you or your loved one had been struggling with a food addiction, you may understand the implications this may have on the various aspects of your life. If food addiction is left untreated, it can rapidly begin consuming your life, creating damaging and chronic symptoms. Understanding how this may affect the different aspects of your life may encourage you to get the help you need . The following are some of the effects of an addiction to food:

Physical Effects

Food addiction can result in many negative physical consequences on the body as an excess of food is consumed. These are some physical effects that may be experienced:

*Heart disease
*Diabetes
*Digestive Problems
*Malnutrition
*Obesity
*Chronic fatigue
*Chronic pain
*Sleep disorders
*Reduced sex drive
*Headaches
*Lethargy
*Arthritis
*Stroke
*Kidney/Liver Disease

.

*Osteoporosis
*Psychological Effects
An addiction to food can be debilitating to mental health, especially if there is lack of support or adequate help. Some of the psychological effects that may be experienced include:

*Low self-esteem
*Depression
*Panic attacks
*Increased feelings of anxiety
*Feeling sad, hopeless, or in despair
*Increased irritability, especially if access to desired food is restricted
*Emotional detachment or numbness
*Suicidal ideation
Finally, food addiction can have an impact on your social life and relationships. Social effects of food addiction include:

*Reduced performance at work or school
*Isolation from loved ones
*Division and conflict within family units

.

*Lack of enjoyment in hobbies or activities once enjoyed
*Avoidance of social events or functions
*Risk of ruining finances or career

How Is Food Addiction Different from Eating Disorders?

Understanding the differences between food addictions and an eating disorder. We will also look at what eating disorders are. Eating disorders are identified into categories, specifically

Anorexia Nervosa
Bulimia Nervosa
Binge Eating Disorder
Eating disorders include both psychological, behavioral, and physiological symptoms. According to the National Institute of Mental Health (MHNIMH), eating disorders are defined as a potentially fatal illness that causes severe disturbances to a person's eating behaviors.

Obsessions with food, body weight, and shape can also be a part of an eating disorder. Anorexia Nervosa is an eating disorder that includes extremely restrictive eating, extreme thinness, and a relentless pursuit of thinness and unwillingness to maintain a normal or healthy weight.

Anorexics typically have an intense fear of gaining weight, a distorted body image, and low self esteem that is influenced by perceptions of body weight and shape. Physical symptoms can include osteopenia or osteoporosis, anemia, brittle hair and nails, lanugo in severe malnutrition, low blood pressure, and heart rate, potential brain damage, and periods of time without a menstrual cycle (in females), or delay or absence of puberty in both males and females.

Bulimia Nervosa is defined as recurrent and frequent episodes of binging with lack of control or perception of lack of control, over binging episodes. The binge eating is typically followed with compensating behaviors, such as

.

Purging
Excessive exercise
Laxative abuse
Fasting
Or a combination of behaviors.
Individuals with bulimia tend to have a healthy or relatively healthy body weight compared to those with anorexia. Symptoms typically include:

Inflamed or sore throat
Swollen glands in neck and jaw
Eroded tooth enamel and sensitivity
Acid reflux and GI distress
Dehydration, and electrolyte imbalance.
Binge eating is when individuals feel a loss of control over their eating, with periods of binge eating that are not followed by compensatory behaviors. Typically those who binge eat struggle with obesity or being overweight.

Symptoms include eating large amounts of food in a 2 hour period, eating when not hungry,

.

eating significantly fast, and eating until uncomfortably full. Those who binge eat, typically do so in secret, may engage in various dieting behaviors without success, and may have separate financial accounts or money for binging, and state feelings of distress, shame and guilt around binging.

In conclusion, eating disorders and food addictions vary considerably. Even though food addictions seem to be similar to binge eating, food addictions are more related to eating patterns and pleasure and reward. Eating disorders are a psychological disorder that are both environmental and genetic in nature.

Chapter 3

How our unhealthy food is making us sick

INTRODUCTION

The world is currently experiencing an obesity epidemic, which puts people at risk for chronic diseases like heart disease and diabetes. Junk food can contribute to obesity and yet it is becoming a part of our everyday lives because of our fast-paced lifestyles. Life can be exhausting when you are juggling school, sport, and hanging with friends and family! Junk food companies make food convenient, tasty, and affordable, so it has largely replaced preparing and eating healthy homemade meals. Junk foods include foods like burgers, fried chicken, and pizza from fast-food restaurants, as well as packaged foods like chips, biscuits, and ice-cream, sugar-sweetened beverages like soda, fatty meats like bacon, sugary cereals, and frozen ready meals like lasagne. These are typically highly processed foods, meaning several steps were involved in making the food, with a focus on making them tasty and thus easy to overeat. Unfortunately, junk foods provide lots of calories and energy, but little of the vital nutrients our bodies need to grow and be healthy, like proteins, vitamins, minerals, and fiber. According to the dietary guidelines of Australian and many other countries, these five food groups are grains and cereals, vegetables and legumes, fruits, dairy and dairy alternatives, and meat and meat alternatives.

Young people are usually the targets of sneaky advertising tactics used by junk food companies, which show out the people we look up to promoting junk foods. Elite athletes like cricket players are not fuelling their bodies with fried chicken, burgers, and fries! A study showed that adolescents aged 12–17 years view over 14.4 million food advertisements in a single year on popular websites, with cakes, cookies, and ice cream being the most frequently advertised products. Another study examining YouTube videos popular amongst children reported that

38% of all ads involved a food or beverage and 56% of those food ads were for junk foods .

WHAT HAPPENS TO OUR BODIES SHORTLY AFTER WE EAT JUNK FOODS?

Food is made up of three major nutrients: carbohydrates, proteins, and fats. There are also vitamins and minerals in food that support good health, growth, and development. Getting adequate nutrition is very important during our teenage years. However, when we eat junk foods, we are taking in high amounts of carbohydrates, proteins, and fats, which are quickly absorbed by the body.

Let us take the example of eating a hamburger. A burger typically contains carbohydrates from the bun, proteins and fats from the beef patty, and fats from the cheese and sauce. On average, a burger from a fast-food chain contains 36–40% of your daily energy needs and this does not account for any chips or drinks consumed with it. This is a large amount of food for the body to digest—not good if you are about to hit the cricket pitch!

LONG-TERM IMPACTS OF JUNK FOODS

If we eat mostly junk foods over many weeks, months, or years, there can be several long-term impacts on health . For example, high saturated fat intake is strongly associated with high levels of bad cholesterol in the blood, which can be a sign of heart disease. Respected research studies found that young people who eat only small amounts of saturated fat have lower total cholesterol levels.

Constant consumption of junk foods can also increase the risk of diseases such as hypertension and stroke. Hypertension is also known as high blood pressure and a stroke is a damage to the brain from reduced blood supply, which prevents the brain from receiving the adequate amount of oxygen and nutrients it needs to survive. Hypertension and stroke can occur because of

.

the high amounts of cholesterol and salt in junk foods.

Junk foods can also trigger the "happy hormone," dopamine, to be released in the brain, making us feel good when we eat these foods. This can lead us to wanting more junk food to get that same happy feeling again. Other long-term effects of eating too much junk food include tooth decay and constipation. Soft drinks, for example,can cause tooth decay due to high amounts of sugar and acid that can weaken the protective tooth enamel. Junk foods are typically low in fiber too, which has negative consequences for gut health in the long term. Fiber forms the bulk of our poop and without it, it can be hard to poop!

Why Do I Feel Sick After Eating Junk Food?

Junk food and why it makes you feel sick (simple breakdown)

To understand better why junk food makes you feel sick, it's important to understand how our

.

bodies use carbohydrates to provide energy to our brain, muscles, and the rest of our body.

Carbohydrates, blood sugar, and its effect on our body

When we consume carbohydrates our body breaks down the digestible carbs into sugar, that sugar then enters the bloodstream. This causes blood sugar levels to increase.

When blood sugar levels increase it alters our pancreas to create insulin. Insulin is what actually tells our cells to use that blood sugar for energy and storage.

When our cells start using the sugar in our blood, our blood sugar levels decrease a great deal. The drop in blood sugar signals the pancreas to begin making glucagon. Glucagon is the hormone that tells our liver to start releasing stored sugar.

.

This relationship between insulin and glucagon is what ensures our body has a constant and balanced supply of blood sugar which is energy.

Now that you have an understanding of how our body uses carbohydrates, it's important to understand how the type of carbohydrates we eat can positively or negatively impact our body.

Different type of carbohydrates (and which ones to avoid)

All carbohydrates are not created equally. There are different kinds of carbohydrates (simple and complex). The type of carbs you're consuming will have a bTreatment: on how those carbs are utilized by the body.

The main difference between the two is how quickly our body accepts and digests them. One is much more likely to make you feel sick.

Simple carbohydrates:

Simple carbohydrates are carbohydrates with a very basic molecular structure. They consist of either a single monosaccharide or two monosaccharides linked together.

Simple carbs are digested and utilized by the body quickly. Due to how quickly they're digested, spikes in blood sugar are very common.

As mentioned previously, spikes in blood sugar lead to severe blood sugar crashes and can leave you feeling fatigued and irritable. This is likely what you're experiencing after eating junk food.

Additionally, any sugar/carbohydrate that isn't used right away is converted to fat. This is why eating foods high in sugar can lead to weight gain.

Some examples of simple carbohydrates are:

Baked goods made from white flour
Candy
Fruit juice
Packaged cereals

.

Table sugar
Corn Syrup
A healthier alternative is complex carbohydrates.

Complex carbohydrates:
Similar to simple carbs, when complex carbs are digested they're broken down and converted into glucose to be used for energy.

However, complex carbohydrates are more difficult (or complex) for the body to break down, therefore they provide longer, more stable energy than its simple carbohydrate counterpart.

Complex carbs usually provide other benefits in addition to the speed at which they're digested, too. Things like vitamins, minerals and fiber are often found in complex carbs.

Fiber, specifically, is an important carbohydrate for our digestive system.

While complex carbohydrates are typically better for you than simple carbs, it's still important to review the overall nutritional profile when determining whether or not to include it in your diet.

Some examples of complex carbohydrates are:

Whole wheat bread
Brown rice
Barley
Quinoa
Legumes (black beans, lentils, etc.)
Starchy vegetables
Regardless of the type of carbohydrates you're eating, it's important to make sure your diet is well-balanced. Over consumption of either type can still leave you feeling sick.

Junk food typically contains large amounts of sugar, or refined carbohydrates, and when eaten cause a spike in blood sugar. The spike in blood sugar is then accompanied by a blood sugar crash which can cause you to feel sick. Symptoms include fatigue, anxiety, irritability, sweating, etc.

The similarities between simple carbohydrates and blood sugar, and between blood sugar and feeling ill, are pretty clear. Fatigue, in particular, is a very common symptom.

There's a long list of other signs and symptoms and issues that come from eating junk food too, some of which can have lifelong consequences.

It's best to eat junk food in the adequate amount which is required to avoid these issues.

.

Chapter 4

What we can do about unhealthy food addiction and overcoming it

*Discipline
Discipline is an important key factor when we need change. If you need to progress in life you need the right amount of discipline.
*Staying around loved ones
There is a saying that goes like this' ' an ideal man is the devil's workshop " so if you are isolated your mind only thinks about the unhealthiest things which include taking in large amounts of junk.
*Exercise
Sports always help your brain to think about productive things.

Food Addiction Help and Treatment

If you or a loved one has found yourself stuck in the wicked cycle of an addiction to food, you have likely experienced a roller coaster of emotions, including despair, frustration, and hopelessness. Living with an addiction to food may be preventing you from enjoying a life you once lived or dreamt of .though the possibility for healing always exists.

By appropriately seeking help and care you can find the resources to address your addiction to food in an effective manner. Thankfully, there are specialized food addiction treatment centers that can help you approach this disorder in a comprehensive manner. Food addiction treatment centers offer multi-specialty treatment that will focus on and address medical issues and nutritional concerns while integrating psychotherapy.

There is also a moderate amount of support groups that you can become involved with, such as Food Addicts Anonymous, Overeaters Anonymous, and Food Addicts in Recovery Anonymous. These groups are 12 step-based programs that effectively address this on the physical, emotional, and spiritual aspects, offering much-needed support to individuals seeking to heal from their addiction to food.

Attempting to deal with your addiction to food alone can possibly further draw you into fear or isolation. Having guidance, help and support from an eating disorder center that treats food addiction, specialist, or support group can provide you or your loved one with the tools and resources you need to recover and heal from an addiction to food.

One way to figure out whether a food is junk food is to think about how processed it is. When we think of foods in their whole and original forms, like a fresh tomato, a grain of rice, or milk extracted from a cow, we can then start to imagine how many steps are involved to transform that whole food into something that is ready-to-eat, tasty, convenient, and has a long shelf life.

For teenagers 13–14 years old, the recommended daily energy intake is 8,200–9,900 kJ/day or

1,960 kcal-2,370 kcal/day for boys and 7,400–8,200 kJ/day or 1,770–1,960 kcal for girls, according to the Australian dietary guidelines. Of course, the more physically active you are, the higher your energy needs. Remember that junk foods are okay to eat occasionally, but they should not make up more than 10% of your daily energy intake. In a day, this may be a simple treat such as a small muffin or a few squares of chocolate. On a weekly basis, this might mean no more than two fast-food meals per week. The remaining 90% of food eaten should be from the five food groups.

Tips to help you lose weight

1. Do not skip breakfast

Skipping breakfast will not help you lose weight. You could miss out on essential nutrients and you may end up snacking more throughout the day because you feel hungry.

2. Eat regular meals

Eating at regular times during the day helps burn calories at a faster rate. It also reduces the temptation to snack on foods high in fat and sugar.

3. Eat plenty of fruit and vegetables
Fruit and veg are low in calories and fat, and high in fiber – 3 essential ingredients for successful weight loss. They also contain plenty of vitamins and minerals.

4. Get more active
Being active is key to losing weight and keeping it off. As well as providing lots of health benefits, exercise can help burn off the excess calories you cannot lose through diet alone.

5. Drink plenty of water
People sometimes confuse thirst with hunger. You can end up consuming extra calories when a glass of water is really what you need.

.

6. Eat high fiber foods

Foods containing lots of fiber can help keep you feeling full, which is perfect for losing weight. Fiber is only found in food from plants, such as fruit and veg, oats, whole grain bread, brown rice and pasta, and beans, peas and lentils.

7. Read food labels

Knowing how to read food labels can help you choose healthier options. Use the calorie information to work out how a particular food fits into your daily calorie allowance on the weight loss plan.

8. Use a smaller plate

Using smaller plates can help you eat smaller portions. By using smaller plates and bowls, you may be able to gradually get used to eating smaller portions without going hungry. It takes about 20 minutes for the stomach to tell the brain it's full, so eat slowly and stop eating before you feel full.

9. Do not ban foods

.

Do not ban any foods from your weight loss plan, especially the ones you like. Banning foods will only make you crave them more. There's no reason you cannot enjoy the occasional treat as long as you stay within your daily calorie allowance.

10. Do not stock junk food

To avoid temptation, do not stock junk food – such as chocolate, biscuits, crisps and sweet fizzy drinks – at home. Instead, opt for healthy snacks, such as fruit, unsalted rice cakes, oat cakes, unsalted or unsweetened popcorn, and fruit juice.

11. Cut down on alcohol

A standard glass of wine can contain as many calories as a piece of chocolate. Over time, drinking too much can easily contribute to weight gain.

12. Plan your meals

Try to plan your breakfast, lunch, dinner and snacks for the week, making sure you stick to

.

your calorie allowance. You may find it helpful to make a weekly shopping list.
Adopt one or more of these simple, painless strategies to help lose weight without going on a "diet":

Eat Breakfast Every Day. One habit that's common to many people who have lost weight and kept it off is eating breakfast every day. "Many people think skipping breakfast is a great way to cut calories, but they usually end up eating more throughout the day, " says Elizabeth Ward, MS, RD, author of The Pocket Idiot's Guide to the New Food Pyramids. "Studies show people who eat breakfast have lower BMIs than breakfast-skippers and perform better, whether at school or in the boardroom." Try a bowl of whole-grain cereal topped with fruit and low-fat dairy for a quick and nutritious start to your day.
Close the Kitchen at Night. Establish a time when you will stop eating so you won't give in to the late-night munchies or mindless snacking while watching television. "Have a cup of tea, suck on a piece of hard candy or enjoy a small

bowl of light ice cream or frozen yogurt if you want something sweet after dinner, but then brush your teeth so you will be less likely to eat or drink anything else," suggests Elaine Magee, MPH, RD, WebMD's "Recipe Doctor" and the author of Comfort Food Makeovers.

Choose Liquid Calories Wisely. Sweetened drinks pile on the calories, but don't reduce hunger like solid foods do. Satisfy your thirst with water, sparkling water with citrus, skim or low-fat milk, or small portions of 100% fruit juice. Try a glass of nutritious and low-calorie vegetable juice to hold you over if you get hungry between meals. Be careful of alcohol calories, which add up quickly. If you tend to drink a glass or two of wine or a cocktail on most days, limiting alcohol to the weekends can be a huge calorie saver.

Eat More Produce. Eating lots of low-calorie, high-volume fruits and vegetables crowds out other foods that are higher in fat and calories. Move the meat off the center of your plate and pile on the vegetables. Or try starting lunch or dinner with a vegetable salad or bowl of broth-based soup, suggests Barbara Rolls, PhD, author of The Volumetrics Eating Plan. The U.S. government's 2005 Dietary Guidelines suggest that adults get 7-13 cups of produce daily. Ward says that's not really so difficult: "Stock your kitchen with plenty of fruits and vegetables and at every meal and snack, include a few servings," she says. "Your diet will be enriched with vitamins, minerals, phytonutrients, fiber, and if you fill up on super-nutritious produce, you won't be reaching for the cookie jar."

Go for the Grain. By substituting whole grains for refined grains like white bread, cakes, cookies, and pretzels, you add much-needed fiber and will fill up faster so you're more likely to eat a reasonable portion. Choose whole-wheat breads and pastas, brown rice, bran flakes, popcorn, and whole-rye crackers.

Control Your Environments. Another simple strategy to help cut calories is to control your environment -- everything from stocking your kitchen with lots of healthy options to choosing the right restaurants. That means avoiding the temptation by staying away from all-you-can-eat restaurants. And when it comes to parties, "eat a healthy snack before so you won't be starving, and be selective when you fill your plate at the buffet," suggests Ward. Before going back for more food, wait at least 15 minutes and have a big glass of water.

Trim Portions. If you did nothing else but reduce your portions by 10%-20%, you would lose weight. Most of the portions served both in restaurants and at home are bigger than you need. Pull out the measuring cups to get a handle on your usual portion sizes, and work on paring them down. Get instant portion control by using small bowls, plates, and cups, says Brian Wansink, PhD, author of Mindless Eating. You won't feel deprived because the food will look plentiful on dainty dishware.

Add More Steps. Get yourself a pedometer and gradually add more steps until you reach 10,000 per day. Throughout the day, do whatever you can to be more active -- pace while you talk on the phone, take the dog out for an extra walk, and march in place during television commercials. Having a pedometer serves as a constant motivator and reminder.

Have Protein at Every Meal and Snack. Adding a source of lean or low-fat protein to each meal and snack will help keep you feeling full longer so you're less likely to overeat. Try low-fat yogurt, small portions of nuts, peanut butter, eggs, beans, or lean meats. Experts also recommend eating small, frequent meals and snacks (every 3-4 hours), to keep your blood sugar levels steady and to avoid overindulging.

Switch to Lighter Alternatives. Whenever you can, use the low-fat versions of salad dressings, mayonnaise, dairy products, and other products. "You can trim calories effortlessly if you use low-fat and lighter products, and if the product is mixed in with other ingredients, no one will ever notice," says Magee. More smart substitutions: Use salsa or hummus as a dip; spread sandwiches with mustard instead of mayo; eat plain roasted sweet potatoes instead of loaded white potatoes; use skim milk instead of cream in your coffee; hold the cheese on sandwiches;

and use a little vinaigrette on your salad instead of piling on the creamy dressing.
In regards to high levels of glucose (sugar) in the bloodstream, water intake is especially important. Lack of water intake has actually been shown to be associated with developing hyperglycemia.

Stop feeling sick and drink some water!

Additional note:

Things to do if you feel sick after eating junk foods

1.Get lots of sleep

Sleep is another great remedy when feeling sick after eating a bunch of junk food. There are so many correlations between sleep and overall health.

Getting a good night's rest has been shown to be associated with weight loss, reduced stress and cortisol levels, and improved overall health.

.

In regards to feeling sick from junk food, quality sleep gives your body the proper time it needs to rid itself of any harmful toxins.

Conversely, consuming high amounts of simple carbohydrates (high glycemic-index carbs) has been shown to adversely affect the quality of sleep we get at night.

So, put the Doritos down and climb into bed!

2.Exercise

There are so many benefits from exercise! Improved blood circulation, stress reduction, better sleep… the list goes on. Exercise is especially beneficial when it comes to our body's ability to digest food.

Additionally, when we exercise it helps circulate nutrients and oxygen to the muscles and tissues throughout our body.

A quick HIIT workout, or even a 30 minute walk, is a great way to work off some of that junk food, keep yourself from feeling lethargic, and avoid feeling sick.

3.Avoid Alcohol

Alcohol is essentially a poison.

When we drink alcohol, especially in excess, our body will metabolize it before utilizing other sources of energy. So, instead of processing all of the junk food we ate, our bodies will be working on the alcohol we drank.

This is counter productive to making yourself feel better…

The first step to feeling better after binging on some junk food is to allow our body to process that food, to digest it.

Not saying you should never drink alcohol again, but its usually best to avoid it if you're

.

feeling sick after eating junk food. Your body will thank you!

6.Be kind to yourself

The last tip I have for helping you feel better after eating junk food is to be kind to yourself. It may sound odd, but it's honestly a really important thing to remember when it comes to the longevity and sustainability of any diet.

It's really easy to be hard on yourself after breaking your diet or binging on some not-so-healthy foods. And, sometimes that can lead to more poor choices or even completely derailing your diet.

If you feel bad, or sick, after eating junk food, start by taking the necessary steps to feel better. Drink plenty of water, get some rest, exercise, etc., etc. But, don't beat yourself up, it's absolutely okay!

One bad meal, or even a few bad meals, isn't going to ruin your progress. What will ruin your progress, though, is thinking you can't get yourself back on track.

Here's my list of the unhealthiest fast food items and substitutions you can make.

1. Soda

soda-alternativesAcidifying, chemical-laden, and loaded with either HFCS or artificial sweeteners (diet varieties), avoid all sodas at all costs. Instead, have some plain water or bring your own.

2. Fried chicken

fried-chicken-and-why-it's-unhealthyMade from conventional chicken laden with hormones and antibiotics, covered with gluten-containing breading and chemicals like MSG and salt, and fried in cheap, rancid oils, fried chicken is high in calories, fat, and other chemicals that can make you sick. Skip it altogether. Please, please just never eat fried chicken.

3. Egg and sausage sandwich

.

egg-and-sausage-sandwichHormones, salt, antibiotics and dairy make that breakfast sandwich a non-healthful choice. Instead, start your day with a Glowing Green Smoothie. You can make several and keep them in your freezer so you can always defrost one and still have one in a bind.

4. Bacon cheeseburger

bacon-cheeseburgerWhere do I begin? Fat, calories, and cholesterol are only part of the problem with bacon cheeseburgers, which also contain HFCS (in the buns and condiments), dairy, salt, hormones, and antibiotics. It's just plain nasty. Instead, opt for a veggie burger or an avocado sandwich.

5. French fries

french-fries-for-lunchFries are simply salty unhealthy fat bombs fried in the worst possible rancid oil. Many fast food places now offer alternatives to fries such as a side salad (no dressing!) .

.

6. Milk shake

vanilla-ice-cream-milk-shakeLoaded with saturated fat, sugar, conventional dairy, and often chemicals for flavoring, milkshakes can leave you feeling sluggish and sick. Skip them and try one of the smoothie recipes in The Beauty Detox Solution,instead.

7. Deep fried cheese sticks

deep-fried-cheese-sticksTake cheese (loaded with fat, salt, hormones and antibiotics), bread it, and deep fry it. How does that even sound as if it might be “food”? Skip them and have some veggie sticks with hummus, instead.

8. Fish and chips

fish-and-chipsMany people select this as a “healthy” alternative in fast food, but it is anything but that. Fish serves as a sponge that mops up all of the toxic chemicals from the sea. Bread it in wheat flour (gluten) and fry it up, and you’re looking at an unhealthy meal. Avoid fish unless you know where it comes from, and opt for a salad instead.

.

9. Pepperoni pizza

pepperoni-pizza-junk-foodCheese and white flour combined with nitrosamine-containing salty processed meats, pizza is toxic and unhealthy. Why not try some brown rice or quinoa pasta with tomato sauce instead?

10. Tuna melt

tuna-melt-sandwichTuna contains mercury, while other additions to the sandwich contain HFCS, dairy, salt, and gluten. Combined with the processed bread it comes on and possibly cheese thrown in the mix, it truly is a toxic horror. How about a veggie wrap, instead?

11. Caesar salad

Caesar-Salad-is-not-a-healthy-choiceThe salad part is okay – it's everything else, the dressing, cheese, and croutons that are a problem. Caesar salad dressing likely contains salt, HFCS, eggs, and lots of fat. Instead, opt for a naked salad and add a squeeze of lemon and some tomato and mashed avocado for dressing.

12. Hamburger chili

hamburger-chiliThe main concern with hamburger chili is the beef, which is very likely laden with hormones and antibiotics. Fast food hamburgers may also contain E. coli and some pretty gross ingredients including artificial color. Instead, have some vegetarian chili or vegetable soup.

13. Nachos

Cheese-And-Chilli-NachosCorn chips loaded with cheese, meat and beans and then dipped in sour cream? Really?? Dairy, hamburger, salt, and GMO corn are just a few of the health issues associated with this high fat, high calorie snack. Instead, have some vegetable sticks dipped in salsa.

14. Popcorn shrimp

popcorn-shrimp-dishShrimp is like other fish, a dirty toxic dumping ground in the ocean for chemicals like PCBs and mercury. Take those chemicals and dip them in flour and salt, and

.

deep fry them and you have a very unhealthy meal, particularly if you dip them in HFCS-laden cocktail or tartar sauce. If you really want fish, try some wild caught Pacific salmon.

15. Churros

mexican-fried-churrosThese sweet bits of dough contain wheat (gluten), sugar, salt, and high-fructose corn syrup. Avoid them and have a piece of fruit.

16. Cheesecake

Cheesecake-sliceDessert in fast food places aren't much better than the main meal. Cheesecake is particularly bad because it not only has sugar, salt, and chemicals, but also hormone-laden dairy. Avoid it, and try some yummy Chia Pudding.

17. Hot dog

hot-dogHave you ever read what's in hotdogs? They are created from "meat trimmings" which may include organs that have been mechanically

.

separated into a paste, blended with salt and other chemicals, and shaped into a hot dog. High in sodium, many hot dogs also contain HFCS and other unhealthy ingredients. Instead, try a veggie sandwich.

18. Teriyaki chicken

Teriyaki-Chicken-bowlMany people believe this is a very healthy option because it is low in fat and calories, but teriyaki chicken contains high levels of sugar, sodium, genetically-modified soy, MSG, and other unhealthy chemicals. Try vegetables and brown rice, instead.

19. Fish filet sandwich

fish-filet-sandwichThese sandwiches have the same problems as fish and chips – mercury and other chemicals, HFCS, breading, and lots of fat. Opt for a salad with some avocado or a sliced veggie burger on top.

20. Beef burrito:

mexican-beef-burritoThe biggest problem in a beef burrito is the beef and cheese. Dairy, hormones, antibiotics – they're all in there. Instead, have a heart veggie burrito with some rice and beans (hold the cheese) if you are hungry.

21. Taco

fast-food-tacoBeef, chemicals in seasonings, cheese, and fried GMO corn all contribute to how unhealthy this food is. Make a taco salad with black beans and salsa, instead.

22. Chicken nuggets

Fried-chicken-nuggetsThe mainstay of children around the world, chicken nuggets are terrible for you. First, they are made from mechanically separated conventional chicken (hormones, antibiotics)and then breaded with flour and salt (gluten), and contain copious amounts of corn bi-products. These are going to harm your kids' health. Instead, offer them almond butter on celery sticks or a hummus sandwich.

23. Milk

.

Many parents select milk for their kids as a healthy fast food choice. Milk is filled with hormones and antibiotics, and is very difficult to digest. Instead, drink plain water.

24. Cold cut sandwich

cold-cut-sandwich-subCold cuts have all kinds of chemicals, lots of sodium, and contaminated animal protein. They are also high in fat, and if you add cheese, dairy. Instead, have a hummus and veggie wrap.

25. Chef's salad

Chef's-Salad-worse-than-a-mealEggs, lunch meat, and fat laden dressing make this "healthy" salad a really unhealthy choice loaded with fat, salt, sugar, and all of the bad stuff that comes in meat. Instead, opt for a hearty green salad with some quinoa or avocado on top.

Summary

In conclusion, we know that junk foods are tasty, affordable, and convenient. This makes it hard to limit the amount of junk food we eat. However, if junk foods become a staple of our diets, there can be negative impacts on our health. We should target high-fiber foods such as whole grains, vegetables, and fruits; meals that have moderate amounts of sugar and salt; and calcium-rich and iron-rich foods. Healthy foods help to build strong bodies and brains. Limiting junk food intake can go a long way in improving our health.

Important note:

Don't rush yourself or let anyone persuade you into doing things you don't want to do, but you have to know that no matter what health is wealth, so you can make the decision and take the baby steps.

Also note that there is no one like you and you are unique and special in your own way

Take care.

www.ingramcontent.com/pod-product-compliance
Lightning Source LLC
LaVergne TN
LVHW050347160826
845677LV00014B/3828

* 9 7 9 8 8 4 6 0 2 0 1 8 4 *